Contents

About the author

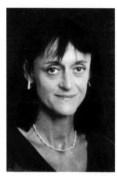

Professor Juliet Compston is Professor of Bone Medicine and Honorary Consultant Physician at the University of Cambridge School of Clinical Medicine and Addenbrooke's Hospital, Cambridge.

Introduction

What is osteoporosis?

We are all familiar with the frailty, fractures, curved back and loss of height that are often regarded as a normal part of ageing. In fact, these are symptoms of a disease, osteoporosis, which can be prevented if steps are taken earlier in life. If allowed to progress without treatment, osteoporosis is one of the leading causes of suffering, disability and death in elderly people. Fortunately, there is now increasing awareness of osteoporosis, among both doctors and the public, and there have been important breakthroughs in its diagnosis and treatment.

Osteoporosis means porosity or thinning of the bones, whatever the cause, and is present in most very elderly people. Bone loss with ageing is a universal phenomenon but becomes a disease when bone mass falls to a level at which fracture (breaking of a bone) is likely to occur.

In normal young adults the bones are strong and break only when there is severe trauma (great external force), for example, in a car accident. With ageing and with certain diseases, the bones become thinner and, as a result, weaker so that they break much more easily. These fragility fractures are the hallmark of osteoporosis and are particularly common in the wrist, spine and hip.

How common is osteoporosis?

The risk of having a fracture as a result of osteoporosis rises steeply with age. At the age of 80 years, one woman in three (33 per cent) and one man in five (20 per cent) can expect to have a hip fracture and a similar proportion will have spinal fractures.

At the age of 50 years, a woman has a 40 per cent chance of having a fracture caused by osteoporosis during the rest of her life; the corresponding risk for a man is around 13 per cent.

In the United Kingdom every year, there are about 250,000 fractures resulting from osteoporosis, of which 60,000 occur in the hip and 50,000 in the wrist.

Although most common in elderly women, osteoporosis can also affect men and may occur at any age from childhood onwards. The frequency of osteoporosis varies widely in different parts of the world, being particularly common in western Europe and the USA, and affecting white European and Asian populations more than black Americans.

As people all over the world are living longer, the number of elderly people in the population will increase dramatically over the next 50 years and this will probably lead to a doubling or more in the number of fractures resulting from osteoporosis.

The consequences of osteoporosis

The suffering and disability caused by fractures resulting from osteoporosis have created a major health problem in many elderly populations throughout the western world; osteoporotic fractures are also an important cause of death in elderly people and 15–20 per cent of people who suffer hip fracture die within six months. The costs to our health services resulting from osteoporosis are enormous.

It has been estimated that we spend just over £2.1 billion each year treating patients with fractures resulting from osteoporosis and these costs are likely to rise steeply as the numbers of elderly people increase.

Case studies
Fred: illness-related osteoporosis

Fred developed Crohn's disease, an inflammation of the bowel, when he was 16 and he required several operations to remove diseased intestine; he also needed steroid treatment. He presented with severe back pain at the age of 22, and an X-ray showed that the bones were thin and one of the bones in the spine (a vertebra) was crushed. A diagnosis of osteoporosis was made and he was given treatment to reduce the pain and to prevent further bone loss. In this case, osteoporosis was the result of a combination of steroids and reduced absorption of nutrients from the diseased bowel.

Mary: postmenopausal osteoporosis

Mary was aged 56 years when she fractured her wrist. She had been well up to that time and had not experienced any previous fractures. The wrist fracture occurred when she tripped while out shopping and fell onto her outstretched hand. She was seen in the accident and emergency department of a local hospital and a plaster was applied to the arm. She was seen a few weeks later by an orthopaedic surgeon to check that the fracture was healing and referred to another department to have a bone density measurement made. The results of this showed that she had osteoporosis and she was advised to start medication to reduce her risk of further fractures. In this case, no predisposing causes for osteoporosis were found and a diagnosis of postmenopausal osteoporosis was made.

Cynthia: premature osteoporosis

Cynthia, aged 70, went to see her doctor because she noticed that she had lost several inches in height over the past year. She had also noticed that her spine had become rounded and that she had lost her figure – her abdomen seemed to have become much rounder and she had lost her waistline. Daily activities, such as housework and shopping, had become increasingly difficult as her back became very uncomfortable after standing for prolonged periods. Although she had generally been healthy in the past, she had experienced an early menopause at the age of 41 years, but she was not advised to take hormone replacement therapy at that time. X-rays showed osteoporosis of the spine. She was treated with physiotherapy and given medication to prevent any further bone loss. In this case, premature menopause is likely to have been a major factor in the development of severe spinal osteoporosis.

KEY POINTS

- Osteoporosis is the result of thinning of the bones, causing them to break more easily than normal

- Although most common in elderly women, osteoporosis also affects men and may occur at any age

- By the age of 80 years, one woman in three and one man in five can expect to have a fracture as a result of osteoporosis

How does osteoporosis develop?

Normal bone structure

Normal bones are composed of a shell of compact or solid bone surrounding connecting plates and rods of bone (spongy bone) within which lies the bone marrow. The thickness of the outer shell of compact bone varies in different parts of the skeleton; for example, it is much greater in the skull and bones of the legs and arms than in the spine. Much of the strength of the skeleton is the result of compact bone but the spongy bone also makes an important contribution. Bone is actually made up mainly of a protein called collagen and bone mineral, which contains calcium.

Bone is alive

Bone is a living tissue which needs to be constantly renewed to keep up its strength. All the time old bone is being broken down and replaced by new stronger bone. If this process, which takes place on the bone

Normal bone

Bones provide shape and support for our bodies. They also serve as storage sites for minerals and blood cells are formed within the marrow.

1. Side view and cross-section of bone (femur).

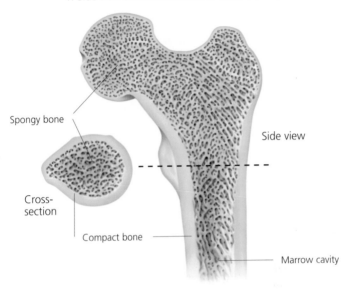

Spongy bone

Side view

Cross-section

Compact bone

Marrow cavity

2. Side view and cross-section of typical vertebra.

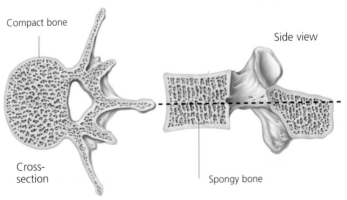

Compact bone

Side view

Cross-section

Spongy bone

The human skeleton

There are about 206 bones in the human skeleton linked to each other by joints. They provide a strong flexible framework that is moved by muscles.

Front view of skeleton.

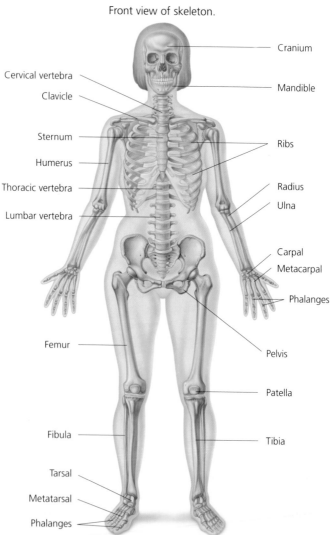

Cranium

Cervical vertebra

Mandible

Clavicle

Sternum

Ribs

Humerus

Thoracic vertebra

Radius

Lumbar vertebra

Ulna

Carpal

Metacarpal

Phalanges

Femur

Pelvis

Patella

Fibula

Tibia

Tarsal

Metatarsal

Phalanges

The human skeleton (contd)

Some bones also surround and protect internal organs such as the lungs and brain.

Side view of skeleton.

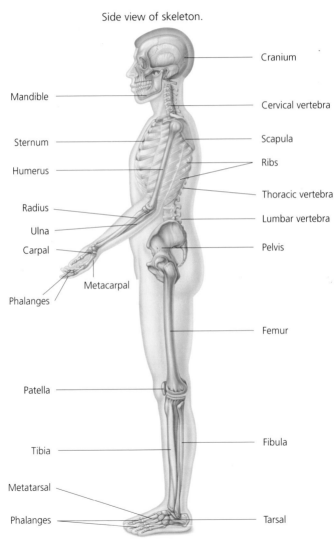

Cranium

Mandible

Cervical vertebra

Sternum

Scapula

Humerus

Ribs

Thoracic vertebra

Radius

Lumbar vertebra

Ulna

Carpal

Pelvis

Phalanges

Metacarpal

Femur

Patella

Tibia

Fibula

Metatarsal

Phalanges

Tarsal

How osteoporosis changes bone structure

Bone consists of an outer layer (called the periosteum) of dense compact bone and a layer of spongy bone. In osteoporosis the two inner layers become much thinner, weakening the bone and greatly increasing the likelihood of fracture.

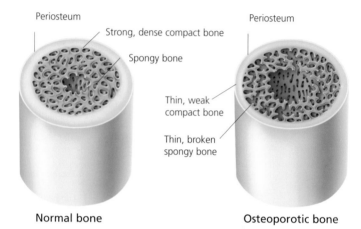

Normal bone

Osteoporotic bone

surface and is called bone remodelling, did not exist our skeleton would begin to suffer from fatigue damage while we were still young! There are two main types of cell in bone: the osteoclasts which destroy bone and the osteoblasts which make new bone. Both of these are formed in the bone marrow.

As we get older the osteoclasts become more active and the osteoblasts less active, so more bone is removed and less formed.

Changes in bone in osteoporosis

In osteoporosis, the amount of both compact and spongy bone is reduced. Thinning of the outer layer of compact bone greatly reduces its strength and increases the likelihood of fracture. As bone loss occurs

The change from healthy to osteoporotic bone

Normal spongy bone tissue.

Strong calcium-rich bone

Spaces between bony material are filled with marrow in living bone

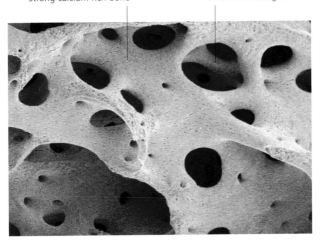

Osteoporotic spongy bone tissue.

Bone mass is lost

Fragile, brittle bone material

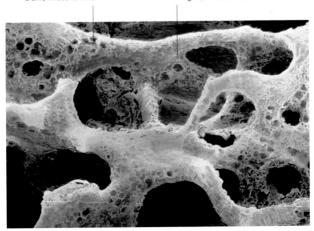

in spongy bone, the thick plates and rods become very thin and the continuity of structure is lost. These changes add to the weakening of the bones caused by thinning of the compact shell around the bone.

Bone mass changes throughout life

During childhood and adolescence, the bones not only grow but also become more solid. By the age of about 25 years, the amount of bone in the skeleton has reached its maximum; this is known as the peak bone mass. Peak bone mass varies quite widely among individuals and is generally higher in men than in women. As would be expected, it is greater in those with a large body frame than in small, slim individuals.

The peak bone mass is very important in determining whether an individual is at risk from osteoporosis later in life. If it is low, then even small amounts of bone loss may result in fracture whereas, if it is high, an individual will be protected from osteoporosis.

What determines peak bone mass?

The factors that determine peak bone mass are not fully understood but there is a strong genetic influence, and calcium intake and physical exercise are also believed to be important. In addition, sex hormones can influence peak bone mass, for example, amenorrhoea (absence of menstrual periods) caused by anorexia nervosa or other illness will result in reduced peak bone mass, whereas there is some evidence that oral contraceptive use may result in a greater peak bone mass.

Age-related bone loss

In both men and women, age-related bone loss begins around the age of 40 years and continues throughout life. In women about 35 per cent of compact bone and 50 per cent of spongy bone in the skeleton are lost during a lifetime, whereas men lose about two-thirds of this amount.

The reason that women lose more bone than men is that, during the menopause, the rate of bone loss increases for a few years. Women:

- have less bone to start with

- lose increased amounts during the menopause

- live longer than men.

Therefore, they are more at risk from osteoporosis. In fact, by the age of 80 years, nearly all women will have such a low bone mass that they are likely to have a fracture if they fall.

The causes of age-related bone loss are not completely understood but oestrogen deficiency is known to be mainly responsible for menopausal bone loss in women.

In many individuals, age-related bone loss is sufficient to result in osteoporosis in old age. In some cases, however, other factors increase bone loss over and above that which would normally be expected during ageing. These are considered in the next chapter.

KEY POINTS

■ Bone is composed mainly of protein and bone mineral, which contains calcium

■ During childhood and adolescence, the amount of bone in the skeleton increases, reaching a maximum in the 20s

■ From the age of around 40 years, the amount of bone in the skeleton starts to decrease in both women and men; this bone loss then continues throughout life

■ The risk of developing osteoporosis depends on how much bone a person has as a young adult and how quickly she or he loses bone in later life

Who develops osteoporosis?

Anyone may develop osteoporosis, but some people are more at risk than others. In any one individual, the risk of osteoporosis depends on a combination of factors including their age, sex and race. Thus an elderly woman is at much higher risk than a young man and African–Caribbeans are at much lower risk than Asians or white Europeans, regardless of age or sex. Genetic factors are important in determining peak bone mass and may also influence the rate of age-related bone loss.

Finally, in some cases bone loss caused by illness, drugs or lifestyle habits may greatly increase the risk of osteoporosis.

Genetic factors

As osteoporosis is so common, many people have seen its effects in one or more relatives and are concerned that they will inherit the disease. Osteoporosis is to some extent a result of ageing, but affects some people more than others. There is no doubt that there is some genetic influence in osteoporosis, although it is not so strong as in diseases such as cystic fibrosis or haemophilia. The peak bone mass is mostly genetically determined, but other factors become increasingly important in later years and may eventually determine whether or not osteoporosis develops.

Nevertheless, the risk of osteoporosis is increased in people with a very slight body build, which is generally an inherited characteristic. Also, it has been shown that women whose mothers had a hip fracture in old age have twice the normal risk of suffering a hip fracture themselves.

Strong risk factors for osteoporosis
Premature menopause
The menopause is defined as the time when periods stop and usually occurs at about 50 years, although any age from 45 years onwards is considered normal. When the menopause occurs before this, either naturally or as a result of removal of the ovaries, irradiation or cancer chemotherapy, this is considered premature.

Women who have an early menopause are at high risk of osteoporosis and other consequences of oestrogen deficiency such as heart disease.

Amenorrhoea
Amenorrhoea (absence of menstrual periods) before the menopause may occur for a number of reasons. It is common in women with anorexia nervosa (restriction of food intake as a result of fear of becoming bigger) and in women who exercise very vigorously, for example, professional athletes, gymnasts and ballet dancers.

Amenorrhoea also occurs in women who suffer from chronic diseases, for example, some forms of liver disease or inflammation of the bowel. In most of these cases normal menstrual periods have been experienced before amenorrhoea occurs (secondary amenorrhoea).

Strong risk factors for osteoporosis

Certain factors may increase the risk of individuals developing osteoporosis:

- Premature menopause
- Amenorrhoea
- Steroid therapy
- Past history of fracture
- Thyroid disease
- Cancer
- Low body weight
- Others, for example liver, bowel or kidney disease; some forms of cancer

Less commonly, disorders resulting from diseases of the reproductive system result in failure of the production of sex hormones at puberty, leading to delay in starting or complete absence of menstrual periods. Amenorrhoea is associated with low production of the sex hormone, oestrogen, and is a strong risk factor for osteoporosis.

Steroid therapy

Steroid therapy, usually in the form of oral (tablets) prednisolone, is prescribed for many conditions including some rheumatic diseases, some lung diseases, inflammation of the bowel and some forms of cancer. Unfortunately, although steroids are very effective in the treatment of these conditions, they may cause rapid bone loss and lead to osteoporosis. There does not appear to be any 'safe' dose of prednisolone as far as the skeleton is concerned, although the risk of osteoporosis increases with increasing dose.

Short courses of steroids do not have harmful effects on bone, unless they are given very frequently. Steroid creams and ointments applied to the skin, steroid injections into joints and steroid enemas are believed not to lead to bone loss.

Inhaled steroids, which are widely used in asthma, may have small effects on bone but are unlikely to cause problems unless very high doses are used for years.

Past history of fracture

Individuals who have already had one or more osteoporotic fractures have a much higher risk of having fractures in the future. The reason for this is unclear, but it may reflect a more fragile bone structure in those who fracture. This is particularly true for women with one or more spine fractures in whom the risk of further fractures increases about sevenfold. All women with previous fracture, particularly at the wrist or spine, should therefore be considered at high risk of having more fractures in the future.

Thyroid disease

Over-production of the hormone made by the thyroid gland, thyroxine, causes bone loss and may result in osteoporosis if not treated early enough. The same effect may occur if too much thyroxine is used to treat underactivity of the thyroid gland, so it is important that women who are receiving thyroxine should have regular blood tests to check that the dose is correct.

Cancer

Some forms of cancer are associated with rapid destruction of bone, leading to osteoporosis. One of the most common of these is myeloma, which is a malignancy of the bone marrow.

Other risk factors

Several diseases are associated with an increased risk of osteoporosis. These include some forms of chronic liver disease, kidney disease, rheumatoid arthritis and inflammation of the bowel. Some drugs may also increase the risk of osteoporosis, for example long-term use of the anticoagulant, heparin, and some anticonvulsant drugs given for epilepsy. In addition, use of aromatase inhibitors for the treatment of breast cancer is associated with increased risk of osteoporosis, and some drugs used to treat prostate cancer may also have this effect.

Lifestyle risk factors

Many aspects of daily living can affect our bones, including diet, physical activity, alcohol use and tobacco smoking. Although the effect of these on bone mass and fracture risk is generally less than the strong risk factors described earlier, they are important because they can be modified to reduce the risk of osteoporosis.

Diet

There are many factors in the diet that affect the skeleton. A low calcium intake in childhood and adolescence may lead to lower peak bone mass and, later in life, inadequate calcium in the diet may increase bone loss.

Severe vitamin D deficiency, which is often associated with calcium deficiency, causes softening of the bones (osteomalacia). Lesser degrees of vitamin D deficiency, which are common in the older population,

Lifestyle risk factors for osteoporosis

- Dietary factors: calcium and vitamin D deficiency
- Alcohol
- Smoking
- Physical inactivity

increase bone loss and the risk of fracture. High intakes of protein, caffeine and salt may also increase the risk of osteoporosis.

Alcohol

Moderate amounts of alcohol, for example, 14 units weekly in women or 21 units weekly in men, do not appear to be harmful and may even have beneficial effects on bone mass.

However, consumption of excessive amounts of alcohol increases the risk of fracture partly because of reduced bone mass and partly because of the increased risk of falling.

Smoking

Women who smoke have an earlier menopause and lower oestrogen levels than non-smokers. In addition, tobacco is believed to have harmful effects on the cells that make bone (osteoblasts). For these reasons, women who smoke are at increased risk of osteoporosis.

Physical inactivity

Low levels of physical activity in childhood and adolescence may lead to reduced peak bone mass whereas immobilisation at any age leads to rapid bone loss. In elderly people, physical inactivity is often associated with reduced muscle strength and an increased risk of falling and fracture.

Risk factors for falling

Virtually all hip and wrist fractures and some spine fractures occur after falling. With ageing, the frequency of falls increases and there are additional factors that may further increase the risk of falling and having a fracture. Some of these are hazards in the environment, for example uneven paving stones or steps, loose carpet edges. Others are directly related to the health of the individual, for example:

- poor eyesight
- dementia
- physical disability resulting from diseases such as stroke or arthritis
- poor balance
- general muscle weakness.

Alcohol and medications such as sedatives or tranquillisers also increase the risk of falling. Not only do these factors make someone more likely to fall, but they also reduce the normal protective responses to falling, for example putting out a hand to break a fall or regaining balance after tripping. These risk factors for falling are particularly important in elderly people and, when present, greatly increase the risk of hip fracture.

KEY POINTS

- Anybody may develop osteoporosis, but the risk is greatest in elderly women, particularly Asian and white European

- Some of the risk of developing osteoporosis is inherited

- Other factors, such as premature menopause, steroid treatment and anorexia nervosa, greatly increase the risk of osteoporosis

- Bone health is affected by several aspects of daily living, including diet, exercise, smoking and alcohol intake

- An increased risk of falling over, as a result of hazards in the environment or ill-health, greatly increases the likelihood of fracture in elderly people

Symptoms and signs of osteoporosis

What are the symptoms of osteoporosis?

Osteoporosis causes symptoms only when there is a fracture. It is important to realise that bone loss itself does not cause pain or other symptoms; backache, for example, cannot be blamed on low bone mass unless fracture is present. Fractures that result from osteoporosis cause pain and disability; in some cases, the symptoms from these fractures persist throughout life whereas in others they may eventually disappear or improve. Wrist, spine and hip fractures are most common, although fractures in other parts of the skeleton also occur, particularly the pelvis and humerus (upper arm).

Wrist fractures

These are also known as Colles' fractures (after the Irish surgeon who first described them) and are most common in women aged 50–70 years. Typically, they occur after falling forwards from the upright position, the woman putting out her hand to break the fall. They most often affect the radius, one of the bones

Deformity caused by a wrist fracture

Colles' fracture is a fracture of the end of the radius just before the arm meets the wrist. This fracture is common in elderly people with osteoporosis. The bones are usually displaced, giving the wrist a deformity resembling the shape of a dinner fork.

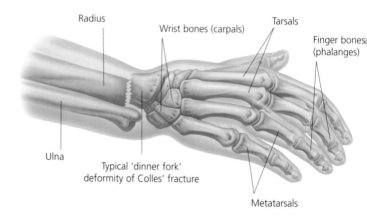

Radius

Wrist bones (carpals)

Tarsals

Finger bones (phalanges)

Ulna

Typical 'dinner fork' deformity of Colles' fracture

Metatarsals

between the elbow and wrist, but are known as wrist fractures because they usually occur near the wrist joint.

Treatment of wrist fractures

Wrist fractures are painful and need treatment at a hospital, generally as an outpatient, although more elderly patients may need to stay in hospital. The fractured ends of the bone are sometimes displaced and have to be manipulated into place before a plaster is put on to keep the wrist still and help the broken bone to unite. Usually, the plaster is kept on for four to six weeks, during which only very limited use of the arm is possible.

Long-term effects of wrist fractures

Although most people who have a wrist fracture eventually return to normal, several problems may arise during recovery. Sometimes the union of the two ends of fractured bone is not perfect, resulting in visible deformity of the wrist. About one-third of women have a condition called algodystrophy after the fracture, which causes pain and tenderness, swelling and stiffness of the hand, and may also affect the circulation to the area. In these patients, there is often persistent pain and stiffness which may last for several years.

Spine (vertebral) fractures
What is a vertebral fracture?

Osteoporotic spine fractures are different from other fractures, in that they do not involve the breaking of a bone but describe a change in the shape of the vertebrae, which are the individual bones that make up the spine.

In the normal spine, the vertebrae are similar to bricks or a stack of boxes. In osteoporosis, bone loss may lead to crushing and compressing, and loss of thickness of the back, middle or front of the vertebrae or a combination of these.

The spine is divided into cervical, thoracic and lumbar regions (see diagram on page 9) containing eight, twelve and five vertebrae respectively. Only the thoracic and lumbar vertebrae are usually affected in osteoporosis, probably because they are subjected to greater weight bearing than the cervical spine.

The vertebrae most commonly affected by osteoporosis are those in the middle of the thoracic spine and the lower thoracic and upper lumbar vertebrae.

How do spine fractures occur?

In osteoporosis, spine fractures may result from falling but more commonly they occur spontaneously or as a result of activities such as coughing, lifting, bending or turning.

Symptoms of spine fractures

The symptoms caused by spine fractures vary greatly; in as many as two-thirds of cases there may be very little or no pain when fracture occurs, whereas others experience severe pain, although the reason for this difference is not known.

When present, the pain is usually felt in the back at the level of the affected vertebra and often spreads round at that level to the front of the body. The pain is often extremely severe and may remain so for days or weeks. In most cases, there is gradual improvement over months or even years; this is variable and, although some affected individuals become pain free after a few months, others may be left with lasting pain or discomfort.

As back pain is such a common symptom in the general population and spinal fractures do not always cause pain, pain in someone with spinal fractures may be the result of other causes such as arthritis or disc problems, which are also very common. It can be difficult to be certain about the cause of pain in some patients, but a useful rule is that spine fractures resulting from osteoporosis do not cause sciatica (pain in the back that radiates down the leg); this is usually caused by disc problems.

Other effects of spine fractures
Height loss

Spine fractures may also cause a number of other distressing symptoms. When several vertebrae are

Effects of vertebral osteoporotic fractures

In this type of fracture the bones do not actually break.
Instead the shape of the individual vertebra changes. The
vertebra becomes weak in the back, middle or front, making
it likely to be crushed and compressed.

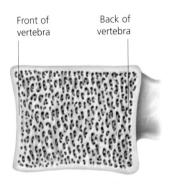

Front of
vertebra

Back of
vertebra

Normal vertebral body – the
side section is more or less
rectangular

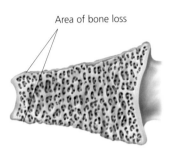

Area of bone loss

Wedging – crushing of the
front causes abnormal
curvature of the spine

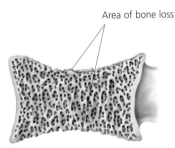

Area of bone loss

Biconcavity: loss of middle
height

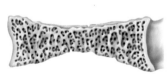

Compression or crushing of a
vertebra arising from bone
loss in the front, middle and
back sections. If several
vertebrae are affected, height
loss may be substantial

affected, there may be obvious loss of height, ranging from one or two inches to as much as six inches or even more. This height loss usually occurs over a period of years. This may be noticed by patients because they cannot reach shelves that they had previously used or they appear to have grown shorter when compared with friends or family.

Curvature of the spine

Height loss is often accompanied by curvature of the spine leading to the 'dowager's hump' or rounding of the back. This change in the shape of the spine causes the chest and abdomen to be pushed downwards, leading to protuberance of the abdomen, loss of the waistline and the appearance of horizontal skin creases across the abdomen.

Physical and psychological problems

The above changes cause severe physical and psychological problems. The combination of pain and spinal deformity often puts limitations on everyday activities such as shopping, housework, gardening and standing or sitting for long periods of time. In very severe cases, the chest is pushed down so far that the lower ribs are in contact with the top of the pelvic bones, causing considerable discomfort.

In addition, there is less room for the lungs to inflate and this may lead to shortness of breath, particularly on exercise. When the spine is very curved the sufferer often finds it difficult to hold the head up; attempts to do so may cause neck pain and headaches.

The change in body shape and its consequences result in loss of self-esteem and often affect social activities. As a result of the loss of waistline and

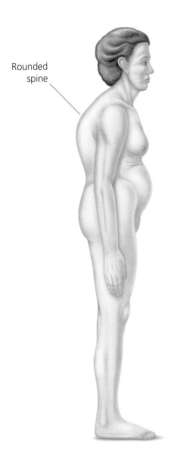

Rounded spine

Height loss and curvature of the spine resulting from osteoporosis can lead to the characteristic 'dowager's hump' – a rounding of the spine.

prominence of the abdomen, many sufferers experience difficulties in finding clothes that fit them; hemlines tend to droop in the front and garments that are shaped at the waist can no longer be worn.

Many patients have a fear of falling which further restricts their physical and social activities; not surprisingly, depression is common in those affected by spinal osteoporosis.

Hip fractures
What are hip fractures?

These are fractures of the top part of the femur or thigh bone. They occur most commonly in much older people, the average age of patients with hip fracture being 80 years. As elderly people tend to lean slightly backwards or sideways when they walk, they are especially likely to fall on the hip, particularly because they often fail to protect themselves by breaking the fall with their arms. Nearly all osteoporotic hip fractures occur after falling from standing height, although very rarely they may happen for no apparent reason.

Surgical treatment of hip fractures

Hip fractures are nearly always painful and require admission to hospital. Surgery is necessary to treat the fracture; if the ends of fractured bone are not displaced the usual treatment is to stabilise the fracture with a metal plate and pins but, if the fracture is displaced (that is, the two broken ends are not lined up together), hip replacement with an artificial joint is often performed. As patients with hip fractures are elderly and often frail, complications of the operation are relatively common and many need to stay in hospital for two to three weeks.

Hip fracture

Elderly people are particularly susceptible to hip fractures in which the head of the femur is broken close to its joint with the pelvis, usually as the result of a fall.

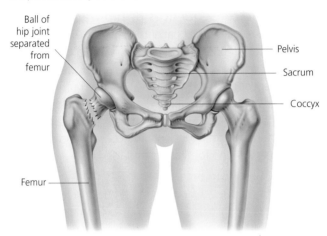

Ball of hip joint separated from femur

Pelvis

Sacrum

Coccyx

Femur

Surgical treatment to repair a hip fracture

Almost all hip fractures require surgical treatment either to stabilise the hip joint with metal plates and pins or to replace the hip joint completely.

Hip joint plated and pinned

Artificial joint

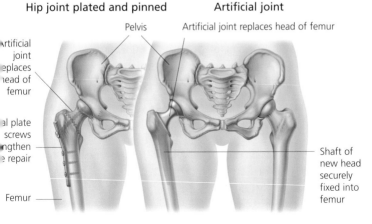

Pelvis

Artificial joint replaces head of femur

Artificial joint replaces head of femur

Metal plate and screws strengthen the repair

Femur

Shaft of new head securely fixed into femur

For a fuller discussion of joint replacement surgery see the Family Doctor book *Hip and Knee Arthritis Surgery*.

Long-term consequences of hip fractures

About 15–20 per cent of patients die within six months of hip fracture. Of those who survive, only about one-quarter regain their former level of activity whereas one-third lose their independence, most of these requiring nursing home care. The remainder are more disabled than before the fracture and many require assistance with daily activities. Hip fractures thus have devastating consequences both for the patient and for families and friends.

KEY POINTS

■ Osteoporosis causes symptoms only if a fracture has occurred

■ Fractures of the wrist, spine and hip are particularly common in osteoporosis

■ Fractures of the wrist and hip require hospital treatment; a surgical operation is necessary for almost all hip fractures

■ Spinal fractures do not involve a break in the bone as other fractures do, but occur when there is compression of the individual bones (vertebrae) that make up the spine

■ Spinal fractures may cause severe pain and lead to height loss, curvature of the spine and other changes in body shape

Diagnosis of osteoporosis

Measurement of bone mass

As osteoporosis is a preventable condition it is extremely important to make a diagnosis as soon as possible. In practice this means detecting low bone mass before a fracture has occurred. There are several ways in which this can be achieved, using machines that measure bone mass – the amount of bone. These measurements are usually made in the parts of the skeleton where a fracture is likely to occur, that is, the spine, hip and wrist.

The reason for measuring bone mass is that it provides information about the likelihood of fracture. Just as blood pressure is often used to predict the risk of stroke, or blood levels of cholesterol to predict the risk of heart disease, so the bone mass in an individual can be used to assess fracture risk.

How is bone mass measured?

There are several different methods that can be used to measure bone mass but the most widely used one is DEXA (dual energy X-ray absorptiometry). This measures bone mass in the hip, spine, wrist or whole skeleton and is often called a bone scan. The value for bone mass produced by the measurement is known as the bone mineral density (BMD) and the general name for tests that measure bone density is bone densitometry.

Bone density measurements on most scan machines can take just a few minutes. Although X-rays are used in making the measurements, the radiation dose is very small, often less than the natural daily background radiation levels. Measurements can therefore be performed in children or pregnant women if required, and can be repeated if necessary.

For measurements of bone mass by bone scan the person is required to lie on a couch. When bone mass is being measured in the spine, a rectangular cushion is placed beneath the thighs (this is done to straighten the lower part of the spine as much as possible during the measurement). A thin metal arm moves up and down over the site of

Bone density measurement

Bone density is measured using a DEXA imaging machine that directs beams of photons or X-rays through the bone, and measures how much energy is absorbed – dense bone absorbs more energy.

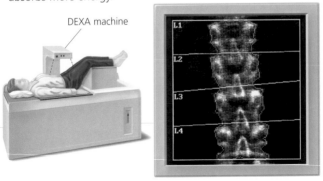

DEXA machine

L1
L2
L3
L4

Monitor image of lumbar spine

measurement but there is no tunnel to pass through as there is in some types of scanning machines. There is no need to undress, although clothing containing metal objects may have to be removed before the scan. Finally, no injections or other unpleasant procedures are involved.

Another way in which bone mass may be measured is by ultrasound, using a method called broadband ultrasound attenuation (BUA). This is usually used for measurements in the heel bone (os calcis) and does not involve any radiation. It cannot be used to diagnose osteoporosis, but a low value may indicate the need to have a DEXA scan, whereas, above a certain value, osteoporosis is very unlikely.

X-rays

X-rays, in a routine radiology department, are used to diagnose fractures in osteoporosis. They are not, however, very useful in detecting low bone mass because the density

X-ray imaging

X-ray images are useful for determining bone fractures, but are not of much value in diagnosing osteoporosis.

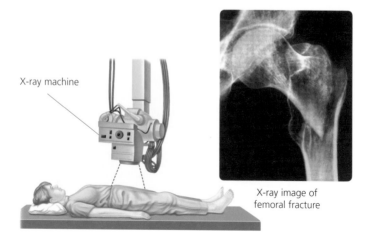

X-ray machine

X-ray image of femoral fracture

of the bones on an X-ray depends on a number of technical factors to do with the X-ray itself, as well as the actual amount of bone present. It is thought that low bone mass can be seen reliably on an X-ray only when the bones have become half their normal density! Thin bones on an X-ray should therefore be taken seriously but, conversely, low bone mass will often not be detected on an X-ray.

At present, X-rays are the only widely available method for detecting spinal fractures. However, the latest DEXA machines can produce very clear pictures of the spine and may eventually be used instead of X-rays to diagnose spinal fractures. One important advantage of this would be that the radiation dose involved is much lower for DEXA than with ordinary X-rays.

Blood and urine tests

Osteoporosis cannot be diagnosed by blood and urine tests, but these are often used to look for other conditions

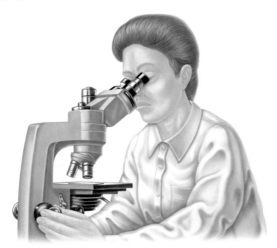

Laboratory analysis of blood and urine samples can provide useful diagnostic information.

that are associated with bone loss, for example an overactive thyroid gland, liver disease or myeloma (malignant condition of the bone marrow). Blood and urine tests can also be used to measure rates of bone loss and are helpful in predicting fracture risk. They may also be used to monitor the response to treatment, although as yet they are not widely used in clinical practice.

Who should be investigated for osteoporosis?
Screening for osteoporosis
At present, bone densitometry is the most accurate way of diagnosing osteoporosis. The question has often been raised as to whether all postmenopausal women should have bone density measurements.

At present, however, experts believe that there is not a place for mass screening for osteoporosis, either in postmenopausal women or in elderly people, although this may change in the future.

Use of risk factors to select for bone density measurements
In the absence of a screening programme, how can those at risk from osteoporosis be selected so that treatment is given before fracture occurs?

The method used by doctors at present is to select for testing people with strong risk factors for osteoporosis, for example those receiving oral steroid therapy or those with amenorrhoea or an early menopause. All these should have a bone density measurement so that it can be established whether treatment is needed to protect the bones.

Use of bone density measurement to confirm a diagnosis of osteoporosis

In individuals who have already had one or more fractures, bone density measurements are often used to establish whether the fractures are the result of osteoporosis; sometimes, for example, in patients with many spontaneous spine fractures, this may be obvious but in some cases it can be hard to distinguish fragility fractures from those caused by trauma (excessive force).

Bone density measurements are also performed in people found to have signs suggestive of osteoporosis, for example, height loss or thin bones on X-ray, to ensure that a correct diagnosis is made. Some degree of height loss with ageing is normal (usually an inch or couple of centimetres or so); however, height loss of two inches (about five centimetres) or more may indicate the presence of osteoporosis although other diseases, particularly osteoarthritis, may be responsible.

Use of bone density to assess the effects of treatment

Bone density measurements are used to assess the effects of treatment given for osteoporosis. However, many doctors now believe that routine monitoring is unnecessary because very few individuals fail to respond to treatment; instead, it may be more useful to assess bone density after about five years of therapy to establish whether treatment should be continued.

Thinning of the bones on X-rays

Doctors may sometimes comment that the bones appear 'thin' on an X-ray. Quite often this is a chance finding on an X-ray that has been performed for reasons unrelated to osteoporosis.

When bone densitometry should be used

Individuals who have one or more of the 'Strong risk factors' listed below should visit their doctor and request bone density screening. So, too, should people who have signs suggesting that osteoporosis may already be present.

Strong risk factors:

- Premature menopause
- Amenorrhoea
- Sex hormone deficiency in men
- Steroid therapy (oral)
- Overactive thyroid gland
- Intestinal disease
- Anorexia nervosa
- Severe liver or kidney disease
- Low body weight
- Family history of hip fracture
- Rheumatoid arthritis
- Treatment with aromatase inhibitors

Signs suggesting osteoporosis:

- Thinning of bones on X-ray
- Previous fracture resulting from minor injury
- Height loss

It should always be taken seriously because definite thinning of the bones on X-ray pictures usually means that there has already been considerable bone loss and the risk of fracture is therefore likely to be high.

Are bone density measurements widely available?

Unfortunately, bone density measurements are not as widely available as they should be and, in some parts of the UK, it is very difficult or even impossible for general practitioners and hospital doctors to obtain bone densitometry for their patients.

It is very important that bone density services are provided by experts, because running the machines, interpretation of the results and providing advice on treatment all require training and experience. The best units are generally based in hospitals and involve one or more consultant physicians with expertise in bone disease.

If bone density measurements are not available, doctors may have to base their decisions about treatment on the presence of risk factors. This is the best option in the circumstances but is far from ideal and is likely to result in unnecessary treatment for some people, because not everyone with a strong risk factor will actually have osteoporosis.

KEY POINTS

- The amount of bone (bone mass) can be measured in different parts of the skeleton; the most widely used method is DEXA

- These bone scans can be used to predict the risk of fractures in an individual

- Ordinary X-rays are used to detect fractures, and blood and urine tests are performed to check for other illnesses that predispose to osteoporosis

- There is no screening programme available for osteoporosis in healthy women; however, bone scans are advised in people with strong risk factors, for example oral steroid treatment, sex hormone deficiency or a past history of fractures

Treatment of osteoporosis: general measures

General considerations

Treatment of osteoporosis involves:

- relief of pain
- improving mobility
- helping to cope with the psychosocial effects of the disease
- preventing further bone loss so that the fracture risk is reduced.

Although drug treatment is usually necessary to prevent bone loss, there are a number of self-help measures that can be taken by the patient to reduce progression of the disease.

The value of patient education

Most people with osteoporosis find it helpful to learn about the disease and are reassured to find that much can be done, both to prevent further bone loss and fractures, and to treat existing symptoms. Knowing that there are measures that they can take themselves to improve their condition, such as exercise, changes in diet and avoiding falls, helps those who are affected to feel that they have some control over the disease and can improve their chances of recovery. Many people also find it helpful to talk to other sufferers and to realise that they are not alone in having osteoporosis. Patient support groups, such as the National Osteoporosis Society, provide an important source of information about all aspects of the disease and supply a means by which patients can meet each other and professionals involved in the management of osteoporosis. See 'Useful information' on page 91.

Management of pain
How severe is pain in osteoporosis?
Pain is very variable in osteoporosis; some affected people have severe chronic pain whereas others have only minor discomfort. The pain that occurs after hip or wrist fracture usually improves rapidly after surgery, although pain-killers may be required for some time afterwards.

In patients who develop algodystrophy after wrist fracture, physiotherapy may provide some pain relief and improve mobility. In very severe cases a procedure called sympathectomy may be advised, in which nerves supplying the affected arm are either cut by surgery or anaesthetised using drugs. Another treatment that has been used is transcutaneous electrical nerve stimulation (TENS), which is described in more detail on page 46.

Treatment of severe pain
In patients who have acute spinal fractures, the pain may be extremely severe and is difficult to treat. A

period of bed rest may be necessary, although this should be restricted to as short a time as possible because immobilisation can itself directly cause further bone loss. Spinal corsets sometimes provide some relief, although most doctors discourage their use because they immobilise the spine and increase bone loss.

Very strong pain-killers may be required in the early stages after fracture, for example morphine-related drugs. Unfortunately these and other strong pain-killers often have side effects such as drowsiness, constipation and mental confusion, and may also increase the risk of the patient falling once levels of activity increase.

In those with severe pain that cannot be controlled by pain-killers, treatment with a hormone called calcitonin is sometimes very effective. This hormone is produced by the thyroid gland (but is quite different from thyroxine) and has pain-relieving properties which can be very useful when other approaches have failed. Calcitonin can be given by nasal spray or injection. It may cause side effects, particularly nausea and flushing when the injection is given, the nausea sometimes lasting for several hours. Vomiting and diarrhoea may also occur and there may be pain at the site of the injection. Nevertheless, worthwhile relief of pain is obtained in many patients, generally within a week or two of starting treatment.

Pain-killing tablets

Once the pain starts to improve, many patients find that pain-killers such as paracetamol or codeine, or combinations of these, such as co-dydramol, co-codamol or co-proxamol, provide sufficient pain relief to enable daily activities to be resumed. In some cases, non-steroidal anti-inflammatory agents such as ibuprofen are effective.

Individuals react differently to pain-killers, as far as both their effectiveness and their side effects are concerned, so it is worth trying different preparations if the one prescribed is not very effective. There are many different pain-killers available from the chemist or by prescription and it may take a while to find the best one, but it is worth persisting.

Other measures

A number of other measures may also provide pain relief. Heat pads, hot water bottles and icepacks may reduce pain. Some patients find that acupuncture is effective, although this is not generally available on the National Health Service.

TENS (transcutaneous electrical nerve stimulation) also helps to relieve pain in some sufferers. This consists of a small machine that hooks onto a belt around the waist and contains small electrodes that are placed on the area affected by pain and cause a tingling sensation. The idea behind this is that the

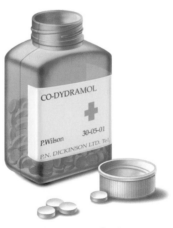

Management of pain.

sensations produced by the machine 'block out' the pain caused by spinal fracture.

Finally, attention to details such as comfortable chairs, with lumbar support cushions if needed, and a suitably firm bed are important and can improve daily quality of life.

Physiotherapy and hydrotherapy

Physiotherapy, that is the treatment of the symptoms of a disease by means of exercise, is very important in the management of osteoporosis and is used to relieve pain and improve mobility. In patients with spinal fractures, the muscles around the spine often go into spasm as a result of the pain, and in doing so they

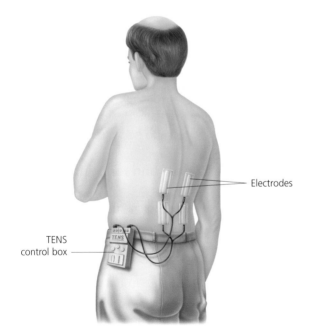

Electrodes

TENS
control box

Use of TENS apparatus for pain relief.

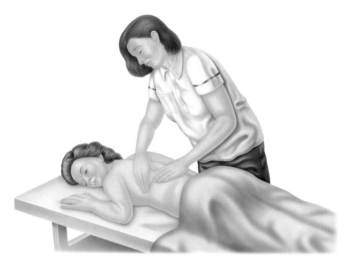

Physiotherapy.

actually cause more pain. Relief of this muscle spasm by gentle physiotherapy which relaxes the muscles will therefore help to reduce pain. Hydrotherapy (gentle exercise in warm water) also helps to relax the muscles.

Restoring confidence and reducing the risk of falls

Many patients with osteoporosis become very inactive, partly as a result of their pain but also because they lose confidence and are frightened that they will fall and have another fracture, or that exercise may lead to further damage of the bones in the spine. Physiotherapy and hydrotherapy can be very helpful in improving mobility and restoring confidence in such people. They also improve muscle strength and help people to protect themselves against injury if they do trip or fall.

Effects on posture

Another useful effect of physiotherapy is that it can improve posture. The presence of back pain and muscle spasm often makes the sufferer tend to round the shoulders and avoid straightening the back, but with gentle exercises and relaxation of the spine muscles posture will often improve. Patients with spinal osteoporosis are understandably distressed by the change in the shape of their spine and the rounding of the back that occurs and it is important to realise that this can often be improved.

What exercises are best?

The amount and type of exercise that should be undertaken will vary according to how severely the individual is affected. Over-vigorous exercise can be harmful in some circumstances so it is best to seek advice, from either a doctor or physiotherapist, before starting exercises (see page 57).

In general, exercises that cause pain should be avoided although a little discomfort can be ignored. The National Osteoporosis Society (page 94) has produced a booklet on exercises for osteoporosis sufferers which many patients find helpful.

KEY POINTS

■ Pain can be very severe in osteoporosis and strong pain-killers may be necessary in the early stages after fracture

■ Injections of a hormone called calcitonin may help to relieve severe pain after spinal fractures

■ Other helpful measures include physiotherapy, hydrotherapy and TENS

Self-help measures

The importance of self-help

As mentioned earlier, there are a number of lifestyle factors that affect bone mass and for many of these an individual can take measures to improve the health of their bones. Many people find that by adopting self-help measures they feel more in control of the disease and are able to make their own contribution to improvement or recovery. These measures are just as important in people who do not have osteoporosis, because they will reduce the risk of developing the disease.

Food and nutrition
Calcium

A balanced diet is very important for the bones. In particular, an adequate calcium intake will help to achieve a good peak bone mass and will also reduce age-related bone loss later in life. Although many foods contain calcium, not all of these actually release much calcium into the body after they have been eaten and the best source of calcium in the diet is dairy produce, for example milk and cheese.

Most experts believe that about one gram of calcium should be taken in the diet each day; one pint of milk contains about three-quarters of this amount

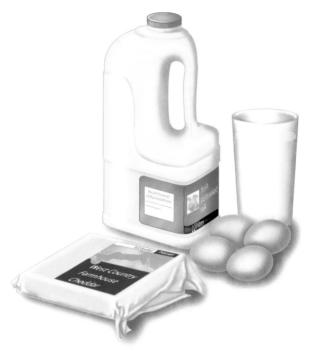

A balanced diet, rich in calcium, will help you to achieve and maintain good bone mass.

(including skimmed milk, which actually contains a little more calcium than full cream or semi-skimmed milk).

Unfortunately, some people are unable to tolerate dairy products and it may be necessary for them to have calcium supplements, because it is very difficult to manage to consume one gram of calcium each day without using dairy products.

There is a bewildering choice of calcium products on sale in health food shops and chemists. These contain different amounts of calcium and, in many instances, are insufficient to protect the bones against osteoporosis.

Dietary sources of calcium

Most experts believe that about 1 gram of calcium should be taken in the diet each day (1 gram = 1,000 milligrams).

Dairy products (average portion)	Calcium (milligrams or mg)
Skimmed milk: 190 millilitres or ml (third of a pint)	235
Semi-skimmed milk: 190 ml (third of a pint)	231
Whole milk: 190 ml (third of a pint)	224
Yoghurt: 140 g (5 oz)	240
Edam cheese: 30 g (1 oz)	216
Cheddar cheese: 30 g (1 oz)	207
Cottage cheese: 30 g (1 oz)	82
Non-dairy products (average portion)	**Calcium (mg)**
Tofu (steamed): 100 g	510
Sardines in oil (drained): 60 g	220
Dried figs: 30 g	75
Baked beans: 120 g (4 oz)	50
1 orange	47
1 slice white bread	28
1 slice brown bread	7

It is therefore important to make sure that the preparation chosen contains enough calcium; if in doubt, it is best to ask a pharmacist or your doctor.

Harmful effects of excessive weight loss

Excessive slimming has harmful effects on the bones. Patients with anorexia nervosa often have severe osteoporosis, even though they are young, and, although some of the bone loss is caused by amenorrhoea, their low body weight also plays an important part. Anorexia nervosa often develops during adolescence, when the skeleton should be growing and bone loss at this stage leads to a low peak bone mass and greatly increased risk of osteoporosis. Conversely, people who are overweight tend to have a greater bone mass, but this does not mean that obesity should be encouraged, because it has so many harmful effects on health!

The best course is to aim for a normal weight for height and body build; patients with osteoporosis who are underweight should be encouraged to achieve normal weight if possible.

Are people on special diets at increased risk?

There are probably lots of other substances in the diet that are important for our bones. Other than taking plenty of calcium, however, special diets are not advised for patients with osteoporosis. Vegetarians are sometimes concerned that their diet may increase the risk of osteoporosis. Provided that they have an adequate calcium intake, there is no evidence that being a vegetarian is bad for bones; in fact, eating large amounts of protein, as in meat, may increase the loss of calcium from the body. However, vegetarians who avoid all dairy produce should be advised to take calcium supplements.

What should you weigh?

- The body mass index (BMI) is a useful measure of healthy weight
- Find out your height in metres and weight in kilograms
- Calculate your BMI like this

$$BMI = \frac{\text{Your weight (kg)}}{[\text{Your height (metres)} \times \text{Your height (metres)}]}$$

e.g. $24.8 = \dfrac{70}{[1.68 \times 1.68]}$

- You are recommended to try to maintain a BMI in the range 20–25
- The chart below is an easier way of estimating your BMI. Read off your height and your weight. The point where the lines cross in the chart indicates your BMI

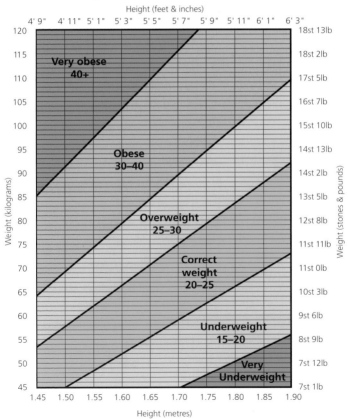

Vitamin D

Deficiency of vitamin D is common in elderly people and can cause bone loss, so it is important to make sure that adequate vitamin D is provided. Vitamin D is made by the skin when exposed to sunlight, and even in the UK this usually provides enough to maintain normal body levels. However, in elderly people who are housebound or go out little or in Muslim women who dress traditionally, vitamin D deficiency often occurs. Vitamin D can be taken in the diet, but the main source is fatty fish such as halibut and mackerel, which many people do not eat regularly. Dairy products contain smaller amounts of vitamin D and a few foods are fortified with the vitamin. For those who do not go out of doors much, dietary intake is often insufficient and supplements are required.

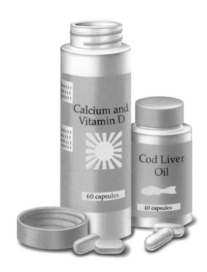

Vitamin D deficiency can cause bone loss. Vitamin D can be taken in the diet or as a supplement.

Chemists and health food shops contain a large number of preparations containing vitamin D, often in combination with other vitamins and minerals. The amount of vitamin D contained in these preparations varies; the recommended daily intake is 400 international units (IU) but in elderly people, 800 IU daily is probably required. In these doses vitamin D is completely safe and has no side effects.

Exercise

Exercise is good for bones, as well as for many other aspects of our health. Complete immobilisation leads to rapid bone loss, whereas weight-bearing exercise can actually increase bone mass, particularly in childhood and adolescence.

In older people, exercise may slow down the bone loss that occurs with ageing and improve general fitness, thus reducing the risk of falling. So, from the point of view of preventing osteoporosis, it is advisable to take exercise at all ages.

What types of exercise are good for bones?

In order to benefit the bones, exercise must be weight bearing and it will affect only those bones that are directly involved in taking the strain. It has been shown that jumping up and down or skipping can increase bone mass in the hips in young women and several studies have shown that brisk walking for 30 minutes or so for three or four days each week may reduce bone loss in the spine and hips in older women. Swimming, although good for relaxing tense muscles, does not benefit bone mass because it does not involve weight bearing.

Over-exercising may be harmful

Very vigorous exercise can actually be harmful to bones, particularly in young women. Some marathon runners, ballet dancers and other sportswomen become amenorrhoeic as a result of excessive exercise and suffer bone loss and fractures. In general, it is best to take moderate exercise and aim for brisk walking for 30 minutes or so on as many days as possible. Use stairs rather than the lift or escalator and use the car only when strictly necessary!

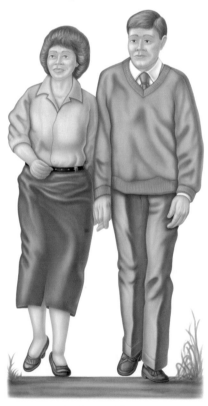

Exercise is good for bones.

Smoking

Smoking is bad for virtually every aspect of health and the bones are no exception. There is also evidence that some treatments for osteoporosis may be less effective in those who smoke than in non-smokers.

Alcohol

Drinking large amounts of alcohol may be harmful to the bones but the good news is that moderate amounts (for example, 14 units weekly for women and 21 units weekly for men) may actually be beneficial! One unit is equivalent to half a pint of beer, a glass of wine or a single measure of spirits and it is best to limit drinking to the above amounts.

Avoiding falls

There are many hazards in the environment that increase the risk of falling and simply being aware of these will help to protect against a fall that could result in fracture. Icy pavements and roads, uneven pavement stones and steep steps are obvious examples where everybody should be careful, but especially those who have osteoporosis. Potential hazards in the home include loose carpets and rugs, slippery floors and loose flexes.

Poor eyesight also increases the risk of falling and can often be improved by a visit to the optician. For those with difficulty in balancing a stick may be helpful, particularly when outside the home.

If in doubt, seek advice

If you are concerned that you may have osteoporosis or are at risk of developing the disease in the future, seek advice from your general practitioner. The earlier the diagnosis is made, the better the outlook. Your doctor may refer you to a hospital specialist, because bone densitometers are usually based in hospitals. Alternatively, he or she may be able to reassure you that you are not at increased risk and put your mind at rest.

Support groups

Many people with osteoporosis find it helpful to talk to other sufferers and in many parts of the country there are local support groups run by the National Osteoporosis Society (NOS; see page 94). The NOS provides booklets on many aspects of osteoporosis that are written for sufferers and provide clear, practical advice. They also run a telephone helpline staffed by specialist osteoporosis nurses and produce a quarterly newsletter for their members.

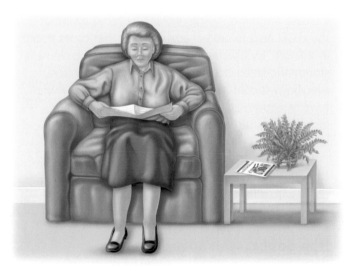

Support groups supply useful services, such as newsletters.

KEY POINTS

■ There are a number of measures that individuals can take to keep their bones in good health and thus reduce their risk of osteoporosis

■ Diet is important, particularly calcium, which is available mainly in the form of milk and other dairy products; vitamin D deficiency should be avoided, particularly in elderly people

■ Exercise is good for the bones at all stages of life

■ Smoking increases the risk of osteoporosis; alcohol in moderation is not harmful

■ Many measures can be taken to reduce the risk of falling and thus decrease the likelihood of fracture

Drugs used in the treatment of osteoporosis

What is the objective of treatment?

Most of the treatments currently licensed for osteoporosis act by preventing bone loss. They reduce the risk of fractures but cannot 'cure' osteoporosis, once this has developed, in the sense of restoring the bones to their previous state. This is why it is best to take preventive or remedial steps as early as possible in people at risk of the disease.

However, treatment is always worthwhile, even in people with severe osteoporosis, because it will reduce the risk of having more fractures. No one with osteoporosis should be refused treatment.

Treatments for osteoporosis have to be taken for a long time

It is important to realise that the drugs used in the treatment of osteoporosis will not have immediate effects on existing symptoms, particularly pain. In addition, once spinal fractures have occurred the shape of the affected vertebrae cannot be restored to normal, so if the spine has become rounded this will not be corrected by the treatment. However, it is now known that treatments work quite rapidly in terms of reducing fractures, with significant benefits as early as six months to one year after starting therapy.

All treatments for osteoporosis have to be taken for several years and, because there is no obvious effect on signs and symptoms of the disease, it may sometimes be tempting to stop taking the treatment or to take it only from time to time. This temptation should be firmly resisted because long-term treatment is required for a full effect on bone loss and fracture rate.

There is now a choice of treatments for osteoporosis and the pros and cons of these should be discussed with your doctor, who will advise which treatment(s) is likely to be most suitable for you. It is very important that you feel happy with your treatment and you should inform your doctor about your preferences. If, after starting treatment, you find that you do not get on well with the drug, you should go to see your doctor because it is likely that he or she will be able to find you another, more suitable treatment. In general, treatments for osteoporosis are prescribed for between five and ten years.

Bisphosphonates

The bisphosphonates are a group of synthetic drugs that are increasingly used in the treatment of osteoporosis. Their main effect is to inactivate the bone-destroying cells, osteoclasts, thus preventing bone loss.

Four bisphosphonates, etidronate, alendronate, risedronate and ibandronate, are currently available for the prevention and treatment of osteoporosis. Of

How bisphosphonates act on bone

Bone is composed of multi-layered tubes called haversian canals. The bone-building osteoblasts and bone-destroying osteoclasts are located between the layers of the haversian canals. Biophosphonates inhibit the action of osteoclasts.

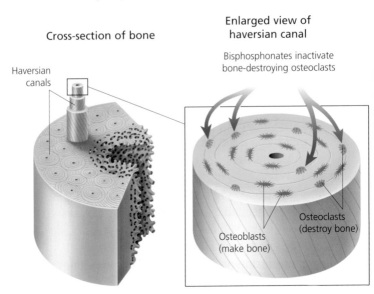

Cross-section of bone

Enlarged view of haversian canal

Bisphosphonates inactivate bone-destroying osteoclasts

Haversian canals

Osteoclasts (destroy bone)

Osteoblasts (make bone)

these, alendronate and risedronate are most widely used and have been shown to reduce fractures in the spine, wrist and hip.

Etidronate

Etidronate was the first bisphosphonate to be used for the treatment of osteoporosis. It is taken in a 90-day cycle with calcium as Didronel PMO (the PMO stands for postmenopausal osteoporosis). The etidronate is given intermittently, two weeks' treatment being followed by 76 days (nearly 11 weeks) of calcium supplements without any etidronate. This cycle of about three months in all is repeated for a minimum of three years and usually longer. Etidronate is taken as a tablet once daily for two weeks of each cycle and the calcium supplement is provided in the form of tablets which are dissolved in water to make a fizzy drink.

Side effects

Didronel PMO is very safe and has few side effects. Nausea and diarrhoea sometimes occur and skin rashes have been reported. Some people do not like the taste of the calcium supplement, but this can be changed to another preparation of calcium if required. As etidronate is absorbed from the intestine into the bloodstream in only very small amounts, it should be taken on an empty stomach at least two hours after the last meal and food should be avoided for the next two hours. It should be taken with a glass of water (not with drinks containing milk, as this prevents it from being absorbed into the body).

Antacids, iron tablets and mineral supplements including calcium should also be avoided during the two hours before and after taking etidronate, as they interfere with its absorption. Most people find it most convenient to take etidronate at night, just before bedtime. The calcium supplement is taken once daily and may be taken at any time of the day.

Who should not take it?

Etidronate should not be taken by women who are pregnant or breast-feeding, or if kidney function is abnormal.

Alendronate

Alendronate (Fosamax) is also a bisphosphonate and acts in a similar way to etidronate. It has been shown to reduce osteoporotic fractures and is taken as a tablet, either 10 milligrams (mg) once daily or 70 mg once weekly. Calcium and vitamin D supplements should also be taken if dietary calcium intake is low or vitamin D deficiency is suspected.

A combined preparation of alendronate (70 mg) and vitamin D (2,800 IU) (Fosavance), taken once weekly, is also available and may be taken without additional calcium and vitamin D supplements, provided that dietary calcium intake is adequate.

Side effects
Side effects with alendronate are rare but include diarrhoea, pain and bloating of the abdomen, and symptoms involving the gullet or oesophagus. The last usually consist of heartburn or indigestion and in a few cases ulcers and inflammation of the oesophagus have been reported.

It is very important to take the alendronate tablets correctly, according to the manufacturers' instructions, because this lowers the risk of oesophageal side effects. The tablets should be swallowed whole with a full glass of water on an empty stomach at least 30 minutes before breakfast (and any other tablets that the patient may also be taking); thereafter, the instructions are to stand or sit upright for at least 30 minutes and not to lie down until after eating breakfast. The tablets should not be taken at bedtime or before getting up in the morning.

Who should not take it?
Alendronate should not be taken by women who are pregnant or breast-feeding and should also be avoided if the kidneys do not function normally. If there is a

history of problems with swallowing or severe indigestion, alendronate should not be taken.

Risedronate

Risedronate (Actonel) is another bisphosphonate and it is given as a tablet once daily (5 mg) or once weekly (35 mg). Calcium and vitamin D supplements should also be taken if dietary calcium intake is low or vitamin D deficiency is suspected.

Risedronate Combi (available in Ireland but not in the UK) is produced as packs of risedronate (5 mg) and calcium carbonate (containing 500 mg calcium). The risedronate is taken once weekly and the calcium on the remaining six days of the week. Vitamin D supplements should also be taken if there is a possibility of vitamin D deficiency.

Side effects

No significant side effects have been found in several large clinical trials. However, because there is a risk of inflammation of the gullet or oesophagus, as may occur with alendronate, there are special instructions for taking the tablets. These are that the tablets should be taken on an empty stomach, at least 30 minutes before the first food and drink of the day, or at least two hours from any food or drink at any other time of day, and at least 30 minutes before going to bed. As with alendronate, the instructions are to stand or sit upright for at least 30 minutes after taking the tablet.

Who should not take it?

Risedronate should not be taken by women who are pregnant or breast-feeding and should also be avoided if the kidneys are not functioning normally.

Ibandronate

Ibandronate (Bonviva) is the most recent bisphosphonate to be approved for use in the treatment of osteoporosis. It is taken as a single tablet once a month (150 mg). Calcium and vitamin D supplements should also be taken if dietary calcium intake is low or vitamin D deficiency is suspected.

Side effects

As with other bisphosphonates, ibandronate may cause inflammation of the gullet or oesophagus. The tablet should be taken on an empty stomach at least an hour before the first food or drink of the day and, thereafter, the instructions are to stand or sit upright for at least an hour after taking the tablet.

Who should not take it?

Ibandronate should not be taken by women who are pregnant or breast-feeding and should also be avoided if the kidneys are not functioning normally.

Which bisphosphonate is the best?

Although all the bisphosphonates act in a similar way, there are some differences between them, and only alendronate and risedronate have been shown to reduce fractures in both the spine and the hip. They are therefore regarded as the first-line choice for treatment of osteoporosis. Ibandronate has the advantage of having to be taken only once a month, although it has not been shown to reduce hip and other non-spinal fractures and is therefore a second choice in most cases.

For how long should bisphosphonates be given?

It is uncertain for exactly how long bisphosphonates

should be given and at present many doctors prescribe them for a period of five to ten years. It is not clear for how long the effects of bisphosphonates on bone persist after treatment is stopped, although recent studies suggest that bone loss occurs within the first year off treatment. If medication is stopped, therefore, bone density measurement is recommended approximately two years later to assess whether further treatment is required.

Raloxifene

Raloxifene (Evista) is licensed for the prevention and treatment of osteoporosis in postmenopausal women. It has been shown to reduce the risk of spinal fractures, but not of fractures of the hip and wrist. It is taken as a tablet once daily. In some ways it acts like oestrogen, but unlike oestrogen it does not cause

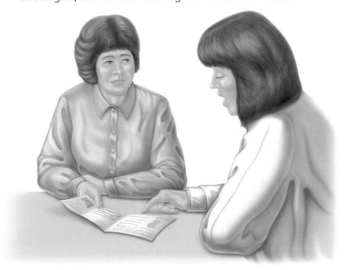

Your doctor will be able to help you choose an appropriate treatment.

vaginal bleeding or increase the risk of breast cancer. In fact there is evidence that it protects women against the development of breast cancer, at least for the first four years or so of treatment.

Raloxifene does not help menopausal symptoms such as hot flushes and night sweats. Its effect, if any, on heart disease, stroke and risk of developing Alzheimer's disease is not known at present.

Side effects

Side effects with raloxifene are uncommon. However, it may cause hot flushes or make existing ones worse, so it is best not to take it if you have menopausal symptoms. It may also cause cramps in the legs and swelling of the legs, although these are not usually severe.

Like HRT, it increases the risk of venous thrombosis and is best avoided in women who have had a previous episode of venous thrombosis or those who have risk factors such as phlebitis (inflammation of a vein), immobility or obesity.

Who should not take raloxifene?

Raloxifene should not be taken by women who are pregnant or breast-feeding, or by women who have endometrial or breast cancer. Unexplained vaginal bleeding should be thoroughly investigated and treated before starting raloxifene. Raloxifene is not suitable for women with severe menopausal symptoms, as it may make these worse.

Hormone replacement therapy

Hormone replacement therapy (HRT) has been used for many years in the prevention and treatment of osteoporosis. It prevents bone loss during and after the menopause and also reduces the risk of spine, wrist and hip fractures. However, because of the increase in the risk of stroke, breast cancer and possibly also coronary heart disease with long-term use of HRT, it is no longer regarded as a front-line option for the treatment of osteoporosis; for this purpose its use is confined to women who have both osteoporosis and menopausal symptoms and those who have undergone a premature menopause. See the Family Doctor book *Understanding the Menopause and HRT*.

Strontium ranelate

Strontium ranelate (Protelos) is a new treatment for osteoporosis. This drug both inhibits bone breakdown and stimulates bone formation, and it has been shown to reduce fractures in the spine and hip. It is taken in the form of granules, which have to be mixed in a glass of water before drinking. It is taken once daily at bedtime, preferably at least two hours after eating. As with other treatments, calcium and vitamin D supplements should be taken as well, unless dietary calcium and vitamin D intakes are adequate.

Side effects

Strontium ranelate is usually well tolerated. Headaches, diarrhoea, nausea and skin rashes may occasionally occur, and there is also a small increase in the risk of venous thrombosis.

Who should not take strontium ranelate?

Strontium ranelate should not be taken by women who are pregnant or breast-feeding. It is not recommended in women with severe kidney disease and should be used cautiously in women with a past history of, or risk factors for, developing venous thrombosis.

Teriparatide

Teriparatide (Forsteo) is another new treatment for osteoporosis. It acts by building new bone and has been shown to reduce fractures in the spine and at other sites. It is given by daily subcutaneous injection, using an injection pen. Patients have to be trained to do this themselves (similar to insulin injections for people with diabetes) and the injections are given into the thigh or abdomen.

Teriparatide is much more expensive than other osteoporosis treatments and is generally advised only for women who have very severe osteoporosis and who are unable to take, or have failed to respond to, other osteoporosis treatments. The duration of treatment with teriparatide is limited to 18 months, but other therapies (for example, bisphosphonates) may be given after it is stopped. As with other treatments, calcium and vitamin D supplements should be taken with teriparatide unless the dietary calcium intake and vitamin D status are adequate.

Side effects

Side effects with teriparatide are uncommon, but nausea, limb pains, headache and dizziness may occur in a few patients.

Who should not take teriparatide?

As mentioned above, the use of teriparatide is restricted to women with very severe osteoporosis who are intolerant of or unresponsive to other treatments. It is contraindicated in women with a high blood calcium level, severe kidney disease, other forms of bone disease or previous radiotherapy to the skeleton. It should not be used by women who are pregnant or breast-feeding and it should be used with caution in women with a history of kidney stones.

Calcitriol

Calcitriol (Rocaltrol) is an active form of vitamin D and has been shown in some studies to reduce the risk of spinal fractures. As it is very powerful, it may lead to high levels of calcium in the blood (hypercalcaemia) and urine (hypercalciuria) which can result in serious problems if not detected. It is therefore necessary to have regular blood checks when taking calcitriol, usually at one and three months after starting treatment and every six months after that.

If high blood and urine levels occur, treatment should be stopped and the calcium levels usually become normal within one to two weeks.

Side effects

Symptoms of high blood levels of calcium include nausea, loss of appetite, vomiting, constipation or diarrhoea, thirst, passing more urine than usual, headaches and excessive tiredness. High levels of calcium in the urine may lead to the formation of kidney stones or deposits of calcium in the kidneys which may eventually result in kidney failure.

Who should take calcitriol?

Most doctors believe that calcitriol should be used only in women who are unable to take other treatments for osteoporosis. First, the evidence that calcitriol reduces fracture risk is weaker than for many other treatments and, second, the need for regular blood tests is seen by some patients and doctors as a disadvantage.

Who should not take calcitriol?

Calcitriol should not be used in people with diseases that cause high blood levels of calcium or in women who are pregnant or breast-feeding. It should be used very cautiously if there is a history of kidney stones or evidence that the kidneys are not functioning normally.

Can calcitriol be used as a vitamin D supplement?

No! Preparations containing vitamin D itself are much safer and provide adequate protection against vitamin D deficiency in healthy people.

Calcitonin

Calcitonin is a hormone produced by the thyroid gland which inactivates the cells that destroy bone, thus preventing bone loss. It prevents bone loss in the spine but may be less effective in other parts of the skeleton such as the hips. Some studies have shown that it reduces fracture risk but not all experts are convinced and it is not widely used for the long-term treatment of osteoporosis.

Administration and side effects

Calcitonin may be given as a nasal spray or by injection. The preparation used is called Salcatonin (because it is made from salmon calcitonin). Side effects of injected calcitonin include nausea and flushing which occur shortly after the injection and are usually transient, although occasionally nausea persists for several hours. Diarrhoea, vomiting and pain at the site of the injection may also occur. With the nasal spray, side effects are uncommon but may include rhinitis (runny nose), flushing, dizziness, and diarrhoea and vomiting.

Anabolic steroids

Anabolic steroids are not the same as the steroids used to treat asthma, rheumatic complaints, bowel disease, etc. They are similar to the male sex hormone testosterone.

Although they are licensed for the treatment of osteoporosis, anabolic steroids are rarely used because of their side effects. The licensed preparation, nandrolone decanoate (Deca-Durabolin), is given by injection every three weeks.

Side effects
Side effects include acne, fluid retention, abnormal liver function and signs of virilisation including hoarseness of the voice and facial hair growth. Most experts believe that there is no longer any place for this treatment in patients with osteoporosis, because other safer alternatives are now available.

Calcium and vitamin D
Calcium and vitamin D are not generally regarded as a treatment for osteoporosis in their own right but are often used with other treatments to maximise their benefits. However, there is evidence that calcium and vitamin D supplements, when used alone in daily doses

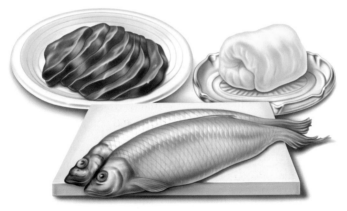

Dietary sources of vitamin D: liver, butter and fish.

How dietary calcium is absorbed into the body

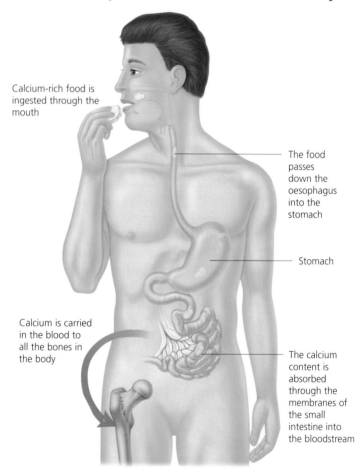

Calcium-rich food is ingested through the mouth

The food passes down the oesophagus into the stomach

Stomach

Calcium is carried in the blood to all the bones in the body

The calcium content is absorbed through the membranes of the small intestine into the bloodstream

of 1,200 mg and 800 IU, respectively, can reduce hip fractures in very elderly women living in sheltered accommodation or nursing homes. There is, therefore, a strong case to be made for giving calcium and vitamin D supplements to all housebound elderly women.

Both calcium and vitamin D are very important for bone health. Vitamin D increases the intestinal absorption of calcium taken in the diet, ensuring that enough calcium gets into the skeleton, which contains about 99 per cent of all the calcium in the body. There are two forms of the vitamin, vitamin D_3 (cholecalciferol), which is made in the skin when it is exposed to sunlight, and vitamin D_2 (ergocalciferol), which is available in limited amounts in the diet. Most individuals obtain their vitamin D from skin production but in older people dietary intake becomes more important.

What calcium and vitamin D preparations are available?

There is a wide range of supplements available, both on prescription and as over-the-counter medicines. For most individuals, a daily dose of one gram of calcium and 400–800 IU of vitamin D is adequate.

A number of supplements contain both calcium and vitamin D; these are often best because vitamin D is required for normal calcium absorption. However, in some situations supplementation with either calcium or vitamin D alone may be appropriate.

Calcium supplements are taken orally as a drink or a tablet and should be taken in divided doses two or three times daily for maximum absorption.

Vitamin D supplements are available as tablets or an injection. Tablets are generally taken once or twice daily whereas injections are usually given once or twice yearly. However, the uptake of vitamin D by the body after injection is often low, so oral treatment is generally preferred. Combined calcium and vitamin D supplements are taken as tablets or drinks, usually twice daily.

Who should have calcium and vitamin D?

Calcium and vitamin D supplements should be given to all women receiving other treatments for osteoporosis unless there is evidence of adequate dietary intake of calcium and they are not at risk of vitamin D deficiency. In the case of calcium, a useful guide is that a pint of milk contains about 750 mg of calcium; if other dairy products or calcium-containing foods are taken in addition to this amount of

Calcium supplements

Calcium supplements are available in a wide variety of formulations. The daily recommended dose is 1 gram (1,000 mg) per day.

Calcium supplement	Dose (milligrams)	Formulation
Adcal	600	Chewable tablets
Calcium gluconate	53	Tablet
Calcium lactate	39	Tablet
Cacit	500	Effervescent tablets
Calcichew	500	Chewable tablets
Calcium-500	500	Tablet
Calcium-Sandoz	108	Syrup
Ostram	1,200	Powder
Sandocal	400	Effervescent tablets
Sandocal 1000	1,000	Effervescent tablets

Amounts of calcium are shown per tablet or dose.

milk, calcium supplements are generally not necessary. Those at high risk of vitamin D deficiency include:

- elderly and housebound people
- some sections of the Asian community
- those taking certain antiepileptic medications
- patients with liver or kidney disease

Combined calcium and vitamin D preparations

A number of supplements contain both calcium and vitamin D. The daily recommended dose is 1 gram (1,000 mg) of calcium and 400–800 IU (international units) of vitamin D.

Preparation	Vitamin D (IU/dose)	Calcium (mg/dose)	Formulation
Calcium and vitamin D	400	97	Chewable tablet
Adcal-D3	400	600	Chewable tablet
Cacit D3	440	500	Granules
Calceos	400	500	Chewable tablet
Calcichew D3	200	500	Chewable tablet
Calcichew D3 Forte	400	500	Chewable tablet
Calfovit D3	800	1,200	Powder

Amounts of calcium and vitamin D are shown per tablet or dose.

- those with intestinal malabsorption (absorption of nutrients from the intestine is abnormal).

Where necessary, it is possible to check for vitamin D deficiency with a blood test.

Side effects of calcium and vitamin D supplements

In the doses described above, side effects are very rare. Nausea, bowel upset (either diarrhoea or constipation) and flatulence may occasionally occur but can often be resolved by changing to another preparation. Calcium and vitamin D supplements are not advised in people who have a high blood calcium level, severe kidney disease or kidney stones.

KEY POINTS

■ Several treatment options are now available for osteoporosis, including the bisphosphonates, alendronate, etidronate, ibandronate and risedronate, raloxifene, strontium ranelate and teriparatide

■ Although HRT is also effective in the treatment of osteoporosis, its long-term use is associated with an increased risk of stroke, breast cancer and possibly also heart disease. It is therefore not a front-line treatment option for osteoporosis

■ Calcium and vitamin D supplements should be taken with these treatments if dietary calcium intake is low or vitamin D deficiency is suspected

■ Calcium and vitamin D supplementation prevents hip fractures in elderly housebound individuals

■ Most treatments are taken for at least five years

Treatment of less common forms of osteoporosis

Most of the treatments licensed for osteoporosis in the UK have been tested only in postmenopausal women and, strictly speaking, are therefore recommended only in the prevention and treatment of postmenopausal osteoporosis. However, there are other causes of osteoporosis that may affect children, premenopausal women and men.

Steroid-induced osteoporosis

One of the most common causes of osteoporosis other than postmenopausal osteoporosis is steroid-induced osteoporosis. There have been a number of studies recently that have investigated whether treatments used for postmenopausal osteoporosis are also effective in patients with steroid-induced osteoporosis. Bisphosphonates have been shown to be effective in the prevention and treatment of steroid-induced osteoporosis and etidronate, alendronate and risedronate are licensed in the UK for this purpose.

Guidelines recommend that individuals taking oral steroids for more than three months if they are over the age of 65 or have had a previous osteoporotic fracture should be given a bisphosphonate at the same time, to prevent bone loss. In others, a bone density measurement should be performed to assess whether treatment to prevent bone loss is required. People who are taking oral steroids should also take calcium and vitamin D supplements.

Osteoporosis in premenopausal women

Osteoporosis in premenopausal women may be caused by a number of conditions, including:

- anorexia nervosa
- over-exercising
- secondary amenorrhoea
- other gynaecological problems.

Hormone replacement is often the treatment of choice in these women because they are known to have hormone deficiency. In this age group, hormones may be given in the form of an oral contraceptive or as HRT preparations.

The choice depends partly on whether the patient wishes to avoid conception, because oral contraceptives are effective in this respect whereas HRT is not.

As the doses of hormones tend to be higher in oral contraceptives than in HRT preparations, patients who are very sensitive to the side effects of hormones often prefer HRT. Finally, the risk of venous thrombosis is probably greater with oral contraceptives than with HRT and this may affect the decision.

Bisphosphonates and pregnancy

Bisphosphonates cross the placenta and are taken up by the fetal skeleton; they should therefore be used with extreme caution in premenopausal women. If these drugs are prescribed, precautions should be taken to avoid pregnancy during treatment and for approximately a year after treatment is stopped.

Osteoporosis in men

For a long time it was thought that osteoporosis was a disease of women and that men were only rarely affected. Recently, it has become clear that osteoporosis affects men quite commonly and possible treatments are just starting to be investigated.

Until the results of these studies are available, it is difficult to be certain about how best to treat osteoporosis in men and doctors have to use knowledge gained from studies in women, which is obviously far from ideal.

Deficiency of the sex hormone, testosterone, is sometimes found in men with osteoporosis. Testosterone has rather similar effects on bone to those of oestrogen and should therefore be replaced if deficiency is shown. It may be given as a tablet, an intramuscular injection or a skin patch.

The bisphosphonate alendronate (Fosamax) has recently been shown to be an effective therapy for osteoporosis in men and is now approved as a treatment at a daily dose of 10 mg. Vitamin D and calcium supplements should be given if required.

KEY POINTS

■ Most treatments available for osteoporosis have been tested only in postmenopausal women

■ Etidronate, alendronate and risedronate are all licensed for the prevention and treatment of steroid-induced osteoporosis

■ Osteoporosis in premenopausal women is usually treated with hormones, either in the form of an oral contraceptive or as HRT

■ Alendronate (Fosamax) has recently been shown to be effective for the treatment of osteoporosis in men; the sex hormone testosterone may also be effective if deficiency is present

Questions
and answers

My mother suffered from osteoporosis in her seventies and eighties. Does that mean that I will inherit the condition?

Osteoporosis is a very common disease which affects one in three women by the age of 80. It is therefore not unusual for someone to have one affected relative, particularly if that relative has lived to an old age and it does not mean that you will automatically inherit the condition. If your mother had a hip fracture in old age, it means that you are at risk from having osteoporosis later in life and should have a bone density measurement to check that your bone mass is normal.

Similarly, if one or more close relatives have had spinal osteoporosis or low trauma fractures, you should also have your bone density checked. If you are uncertain, go and discuss with your GP whether you need to have a bone density test.

I have been told that I have osteoarthritis affecting my spine. Does this mean that I have osteoporosis?

No. Osteoarthritis is a completely different disease which

affects the joints and is not associated with thinning of the bones. It can be distinguished from osteoporosis on a plain X-ray. Osteoarthritis is a very common condition which mainly affects elderly people and causes pain in the affected joints, including in the spine. There is some evidence that people with osteoarthritis are less likely to have osteoporosis and vice versa.

Can the spine fractures that occur in osteoporosis damage the spinal nerves and cause weakness or paralysis?

No. Spinal fractures caused by osteoporosis hardly ever damage the spinal cord or the nerve roots. Back pain that radiates down one or both legs, with or without weakness and altered sensation, is much more likely to be the result of a prolapsed disc or some other cause.

I have breast cancer and am being treated with tamoxifen, which I have been told competes with (antagonises) the actions of oestrogens. Does this mean that tamoxifen therapy will increase my risk of osteoporosis?

No. Tamoxifen is a very effective treatment for breast cancer and acts against oestrogen in the breast tissue. However, it acts rather like oestrogen in bone and protects against bone loss after the menopause, so that it is likely to reduce your risk of osteoporosis.

My mother has severe osteoporosis with spinal fractures and height loss of several inches. Is it too late to give her any treatment?

No. It is never too late to treat osteoporosis, even in very advanced cases. Although there is no treatment that will cure the disease at this stage, there are drugs that will reduce the risk of further fractures in the future.

Do I need to have regular check-ups when I am taking HRT?

Many GPs will see women on HRT at six-monthly or yearly intervals for a general check-up. There is no need to have mammography any more frequently than the three-yearly screening routinely performed in the NHS for women between the ages of 50 and 65 years. If irregular vaginal bleeding occurs and persists after the first three months or so of HRT you should see your GP and you may need to undergo a biopsy of the lining of the uterus.

How do I know if my treatment for osteoporosis is working?

Most treatments work in the vast majority of individuals, so if you take your treatment as advised it is very unlikely that you will not respond. There are no early changes in symptoms to tell you if your treatment is working. Drugs given to prevent bone loss do not affect pain so don't expect any rapid improvement in pain or disability. Biochemical measurements may be used in the early months of treatment to assess response, but are not yet widely available. Alternatively, bone density measurements are sometimes used to monitor treatment but these are only sensitive enough to show changes after two to three years.

Glossary

Algodystrophy: pain, swelling and stiffness which may affect the hand after a wrist fracture.

Amenorrhoea: absence of menstrual periods before the menopause.

Bone mineral density/bone density: the amount of bone or bone mass.

Bone scan: measurement of bone density.

Colles' fracture: fracture of the lower end of the forearm; also called a wrist fracture.

Dowager's hump: curvature of the upper spine.

DEXA: dual energy X-ray absorptiometry. Method used to measure bone density.

Endometrial cancer: cancer of the lining of the womb.

Fracture: a break in a bone.

HRT: hormone replacement therapy.

Hydrotherapy: gentle exercise in warm water.

Hysterectomy: removal of the uterus.

Menopause: cessation of menstrual periods.

Oestrogen: one of the female sex hormones.

Osteoblasts: cells that build new bone.

Osteoclasts: cells that break down bone.

Peak bone mass: the maximum bone mass achieved in young adulthood.

Physiotherapy: exercises to help the symptoms of a disease.

Progesterone: one of the female sex hormones.

Progestogens: hormones often used with oestrogen in HRT.

TENS: transcutaneous electrical nerve stimulation.

Testosterone: the male sex hormone.

Vertebrae: the individual bones that make up the spine.

Useful information

We have included the following organisations because, on preliminary investigation, they may be of use to the reader. However, we do not have first-hand experience of each organisation and so cannot guarantee the organisation's integrity. The reader must therefore exercise his or her own discretion and judgement when making further enquiries.

Age Concern

Astral House, 1268 London Road
London SW16 4ER
Tel: 020 8765 7200
Information line: 0800 009966 (open 8am–7pm, 7 days a week).
Website: www.ageconcern.org.uk

Lots of useful advice, information and fact sheets.

Arthritis Research Campaign

Copeman House, St Mary's Court, St Mary's Gate
Chesterfield, Derby S41 7TD
Tel: 01246 558033
Fax: 01246 558007
Helpline: 0870 850 5000

Email: info@arc.org.uk
Website: www.arc.org.uk

Finances an extensive programme of research and education in a wide range of arthritis and rheumatism problems including back pain. Provides useful booklets explaining the various back problems and ways of coping with them.

Back Care UK
16 Elmtree Road
Teddington, Middx TW11 8ST
Helpline: 0845 130 2904
Tel: 020 8977 5474
Fax: 020 8943 5318
Email: info@backcare.org.uk
Website: www.backcare.org.uk

Offers information and advice for people with back pain. Funds patient-oriented scientific research into the causes, treatment and prevention of back pain. Has local support groups throughout the country with regular meetings.

Benefits Enquiry Line
Tel: 0800 882200
Minicom: 0800 243355
Website: www.dwp.gov.uk
N. Ireland: 0800 220674

Government agency giving information and advice on sickness and disability benefits for people with disabilities and their carers.

British Red Cross
UK Office
44 Moorfields, London EC2Y 9AL
Telephone: 0870 170 7000
Website: www.redcross.org.uk

Provides extra support and care at home, a service offered by volunteers, including: assistance with shopping; collecting prescriptions; companionship; helping to rebuild confidence. The service is available on a short-term basis and is provided free of charge. Referrals are accepted from GPs, primary care trusts, hospitals, social workers and individuals. Contact your local Red Cross branch office for more information.

Gynaecological and Endocrine Service
King's College Hospital, Denmark Hill
London SE5 9RS
Tel: 020 7346 8251
Email: info@kingsc.nhs.uk

Offers assessment and treatment for all aspects of gynaecological problems including the menopause and osteoporosis. Doctor's referral essential.

Help the Aged
207–221 Pentonville Road
London N1 9UZ
Telephone: 0808 800 6565
Email: info@helptheaged.org.uk
Website: www.helptheaged.org.uk

Offers help and advice on many issues relating to older people.

National Institute for Health and Clinical Excellence (NICE)

MidCity Place, 71 High Holborn, London WC1V 6NA
Tel: 020 7067 5800
Fax: 020 7067 5801
Email: nice@nice.nhs.uk
Website: www.nice.org.uk

Provides national guidance on the promotion of good health and the prevention and treatment of ill health. Patient information leaflets are available for each piece of guidance issued.

National Osteoporosis Society

Camerton
Bath, Somerset BA2 0PJ
Tel: 01761 471771
Fax: 01761 471104
Helpline: 0845 450 0230
Email: info@nos.org.uk
Website: www.nos.org.uk

Provides information and advice on all aspects of osteoporosis, the menopause and hormone replacement therapy. Encourages people to take action to protect their bones. Helpline staffed by specially trained nurses. Has local support groups.

NHS Direct

Tel: 0845 4647 (24 hours, 365 days a year)
Website: www.nhsdirect.nhs.uk

Offers confidential health-care advice, information and referral service. A good first port of call for any health advice.

NHS Smoking Helplines

Freephone: 0800 169 0 169 (7am–11pm, 365 days a year)
Pregnancy smoking helpline: 0800 169 9169
(12 noon–9pm, 365 days a year)
Website: www.givingupsmoking.co.uk

Have advice, help and encouragement on giving up
smoking. Specialist advisers available to offer on-going
support to those who genuinely are trying to give up
smoking. Can refer to local branches.

Osteoporosis 2000

Learoyd Way, Hillsborough Barracks, Langsett Road
Sheffield S6 2LR
Tel: 0114 234 4433 (Mon–Fri 10am–4pm)
Email: osteoporosis2000@bt.connect.com

Provides help and information for people with
osteoporosis and their families through their helpline,
literature, drop-in centre and support groups. Runs
exercise for health classes in Sheffield and district.

Prodigy Website

Sowerby Centre for Health Informatics at Newcastle
(SCHIN), Bede House, All Saints Business Centre
Newcastle upon Tyne NE1 2ES
Tel: 0191 243 6100
Fax: 0191 243 6101
Email: prodigy-enquiries@schin.co.uk
Website: www.prodigy.nhs.uk

A website mainly for GPs giving information for
patients listed by disease plus named self-help
organisations.

Quit (Smoking Quitlines)

211 Old Street
London EC1V 9NR
Tel: 0800 002200 (9am–9pm, 365 days a year)
Tel: 020 7251 1551
Fax: 020 7251 1661
Email: info@quit.org.uk
Website: www.quit.org.uk
Scotland: 0800 848484
Wales: 0800 169 0169 (NHS)

Offers individual advice on giving up smoking in English and Asian languages. Talks to schools on smoking and pregnancy and can refer to local support groups. Runs training courses for professionals.

Women's Health Concern Ltd

Whitehall House, 41 Whitehall
London SW1A 2BY
Telephone: 020 7451 1377
Nurse Counselling Service: 0845 123 2319
Email: counselling@womens-health-concern.org
Website: www.womens-health-concern.org

A charity that aims to help educate and support women with their health care, by providing accurate, unbiased information.

Websites

www.balancetraining.org.uk

A research project run by the University of Southampton (email: srn103@soton.ac.uk) offering advice on how to improve your balance system and avoid falls. Visitors complete a short on-screen questionnaire and are provided with an advice pack containing proposed exercises, such as yoga or Pilates, which they can download and follow.

www.bbc.co.uk/health

A helpful website: easy to navigate and offers lots of useful advice and information. Also contains links to other related topics.

The internet as a further source of information

After reading this book, you may feel that you would like further information on the subject. The internet is of course an excellent place to look and there are many websites with useful information about medical disorders, related charities and support groups.

For those who do not have a computer at home some bars and cafes offer facilities for accessing the internet. These are listed in the Yellow Pages under 'Internet Bars and Cafes' and 'Internet Providers'. Your local library offers a similar facility and has staff to help you find the information that you need.

It should always be remembered, however, that the internet is unregulated and anyone is free to set up a website and add information to it. Many websites offer impartial advice and information that has been compiled and checked by qualified medical professionals. Some, on the other hand, are run by commercial organisations with the purpose of promoting their own products. Others still are run by pressure groups, some of which will provide carefully assessed and accurate information whereas others may be suggesting medications or treatments that are not supported by the medical and scientific community.

Unless you know the address of the website you want to visit – for example, www.familydoctor.co.uk – you may find the following guidelines useful when searching the internet for information.

Search engines and other searchable sites

Google (www.google.co.uk) is the most popular search engine used in the UK, followed by Yahoo! (http://uk.yahoo.com) and MSN (www.msn.co.uk). Also popular are the search engine provided by Internet Service Providers such as Tiscali and other sites such as the BBC site (www.bbc.co.uk).

In addition to the search engines that index the whole web, there are also medical sites with search facilities, which act almost like mini-search engines, but cover only medical topics or even a particular area of medicine. Again, it is wise to look at who is responsible for compiling the information offered to ensure that it is impartial and medically accurate. The NHS Direct site (www.nhsdirect.nhs.uk) is an example of a searchable medical site.

Links to many British medical charities can be found at the Association of Medical Research Charities website (www.amrc.org.uk) and at Charity Choice (www.charitychoice.co.uk).

Search phrases

Be specific when entering a search phrase. Searching for information on 'cancer' will return results for many different types of cancer as well as on cancer in general. You may even find sites offering astrological information. More useful results will be returned by using search phrases such as 'lung cancer' and 'treatments for lung cancer'. Both Google and Yahoo! offer an advanced search option that includes the ability to search for the exact phrase, enclosing the search phrase in quotes, that is, 'treatments for lung cancer' will have the same effect. Limiting a search to an exact phrase reduces the number of results returned but it is best to refine a search to an exact match only if you are not getting useful results with a normal search. Adding 'UK' to your search term will bring up mainly British sites, so a good phrase might be 'lung cancer' UK (don't include UK within the quotes).

Always remember the internet is international and unregulated. It holds a wealth of valuable information but individual sites may be biased, out of date or just plain wrong. Family Doctor Publications accepts no responsibility for the content of links published in this series.

Index

Your pages

We have included the following pages because they may help you manage your illness or condition and its treatment.

Before an appointment with a health professional, it can be useful to write down a short list of questions of things that you do not understand, so that you can make sure that you do not forget anything.

Some of the sections may not be relevant to your circumstances.

We are always pleased to receive constructive criticism or suggestions about how to improve the books. You can contact us at:

Email: familydoctor@btinternet.com
Letter: Family Doctor Publications
          PO Box 4664
          Poole
          BH15 1NN

Thank you

Health-care contact details

Name:

Job title:

Place of work:

Tel:

Name:

Job title:

Place of work:

Tel:

Name:

Job title:

Place of work:

Tel:

Name:

Job title:

Place of work:

Tel:

Significant past health events – illnesses/operations/investigations/treatments

Event	Month	Year	Age (at time)

Appointments for health care

Name:

Place:

Date:

Time:

Tel:

Name:

Place:

Date:

Time:

Tel:

Name:

Place:

Date:

Time:

Tel:

Name:

Place:

Date:

Time:

Tel:

Appointments for health care

Name:

Place:

Date:

Time:

Tel:

Name:

Place:

Date:

Time:

Tel:

Name:

Place:

Date:

Time:

Tel:

Name:

Place:

Date:

Time:

Tel:

Current medication(s) prescribed by your doctor

Medicine name:

Purpose:

Frequency & dose:

Start date:

End date:

Medicine name:

Purpose:

Frequency & dose:

Start date:

End date:

Medicine name:

Purpose:

Frequency & dose:

Start date:

End date:

Medicine name:

Purpose:

Frequency & dose:

Start date:

End date:

Other medicines/supplements you are taking, not prescribed by your doctor

Medicine/treatment:

Purpose:

Frequency & dose:

Start date:

End date:

Medicine/treatment:

Purpose:

Frequency & dose:

Start date:

End date:

Medicine/treatment:

Purpose:

Frequency & dose:

Start date:

End date:

Medicine/treatment:

Purpose:

Frequency & dose:

Start date:

End date:

Questions to ask at appointments
(Note: do bear in mind that doctors work under great time pressure, so long lists may not be helpful for either of you)